YOUR KNOWLEDGE HAS VALUE

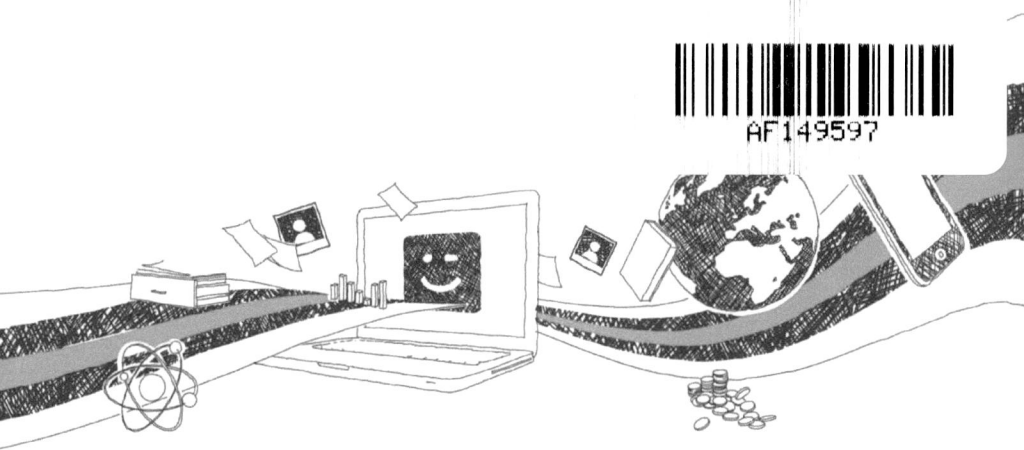
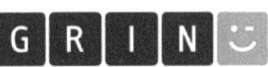

Gichaba Manduku

Towards Achieving the Kenya National HIV/AIDs Communication Strategy

Knowledge and Awareness levels on HIV/AIDS of youths in Secondary Schools - A Case of Eldoret West District

GRIN Publishing

Bibliographic information published by the German National Library:

The German National Library lists this publication in the National Bibliography; detailed bibliographic data are available on the Internet at http://dnb.dnb.de .

Imprint:

Copyright © 2011 GRIN Verlag, Open Publishing GmbH
Print and binding: Books on Demand GmbH, Norderstedt Germany
ISBN: 978-3-640-90445-7

This book at GRIN:

http://www.grin.com/en/e-book/170926/towards-achieving-the-kenya-national-hiv-aids-communication-strategy

GRIN - Your knowledge has value

Since its foundation in 1998, GRIN has specialized in publishing academic texts by students, college teachers and other academics as e-book and printed book. The website www.grin.com is an ideal platform for presenting term papers, final papers, scientific essays, dissertations and specialist books.

Visit us on the internet:

http://www.grin.com/

http://www.facebook.com/grincom

http://www.twitter.com/grin_com

THEME:

A research paper in the area of Hiv/Aids/Communication and
Education

TOPIC:

Towards Achieving the Kenya National HIV/AIDs Communication Strategy:

Knowledge and Awareness levels on HIV/AIDS of youths in Secondary Schools, a

Case of Eldoret West District.

AUTHOR:

By Gichaba Manduku B.Ed, M.Ed, (Ph.D candidate)

Part-time lecturer-University of Eastern Africa, Baraton
P.O Box 2500 ELDORET, Kenya

ABSTRACT

The main objective this study was to find out the level of knowledge and awareness of youths in secondary schools on HIV/AIDs as one of the objectives in achieving the Kenya National HIV/AIDS communication strategy. Adopting a survey design, qualitative techniques, questionnaires, interviews and documentation, a sample of 405 was selected from a target population of 3,854 students. The study was based on a theoretical and conceptual framework with key concepts derived from Harold Lasswel theory of 1948, which has been developed to Modern Communication Theory. The data was analysed thematically. Results indicate that about 399 (99%) of the respondents had heard about AIDS compared to only 4 (1%) who had not. Knowledge had no statistically significant relationship with risk of HIV and AIDS. About 53.3% of the respondents reported to have had sex, with males being more likely to have an early sexual debut. Sexual activity was higher among peri-urban respondents (37%) who also had more than 3 sexual partners. About 71.4% of the respondents were willing to change their behaviour to avoid contracting HIV. On bivariate analysis, exposure to risk factors was dependent on gender ($p < 0.05$), perceived risk and condom used were related ($p < 0.05$).The study concluded that despite their high knowledge and awareness on HIV and AIDS, not all students who were exposed to risk perceived themselves to be at risk. The main preventive method of contracting HIV/AIDS was through condom use, cultural practices like wife inheritance and traditional circumcision increased the risk of infection and that affective communication was not used in schools to reduce HIV/AIDS infection and affection. The study recommended that though creating more awareness on HIV/AIDs was still necessary to diffuse some misconceptions, more effort was needed to address behavior change among the adolescents especially through affective communication. This could be done through inviting specialized groups to speak to adolescents in schools.

Introduction

Background to the study

According to NASCOP (2005) Kenya is still faced with an increasing problem from HIV infection, and the vulnerability of the youth is a key concern. Although HIV occurs in all social and economic classes, much research has concentrated on disadvantaged and deprived communities. This study was carried out among secondary school students for the following reasons: first, adolescents comprise the most sexually active age-group according to Berer and Ray (1993). Statistics indicate that worldwide, the majority of those infected with HIV are between 20 and 45 years. When the slow rate of progression from HIV to AIDS is factored in, then it is highly likely that many of these adults were infected with HIV during their youth (NASCOP, 2005). Second, adolescence is characterized by experimentation with and initiation into risky sexual behavioral practices, including sex, alcohol and drugs. Third, since the present sexual behaviour of the youth will determine the future level of HIV infection, it is crucial to protect the current generation from contracting HIV in order to ensure healthy future generations (CBS, 2004). And lastly, several studies have shown that today's young adults are becoming increasingly sexually active at a tender age. Few of them use contraceptives and are therefore at risk of HIV and AIDS and unwanted pregnancy (Kermyt and Beutel, 2005).

A study conducted by Wong, Chin, Low and Jaafar, assessing the knowledge, attitudes and beliefs about HIV/AIDS among Malaysian adolescents indicated that HIV/AIDS knowledge among the adolescents was moderate and with misconceptions (Wrong et al., 2008). Although knowledge alone does not change behaviour and there is no significant relationship between sexual knowledge and safe sex, knowledge of the facts of HIV transmission plays an obvious role in increasing the likelihood of safer sex through perceptions of individual risk (Tehrani and Afzali, 2008). Adolescents have poor knowledge of preventive sexual practices related to HIV and AIDS (Jara et al., 2008). Even though many adolescents have heard about HIV/AIDS many of them have misconceived ideas on its infection, transmission and prevention. A majority of youths have heard of AIDS, but many do not know its transmission pattern properly or have

3

misconceptions, have not been informed about the preventive effects of condoms and have a low perception of their individual risk (Tehrani and Afzali, 2008). Adolescents' knowledge and its influence' concluded that although adolescents' knowledge of HIV transmission might have improved over the past few years, their risk-related behaviors remain unchanged (Ocran and Danso, 2009).

The objectives of the study were:

1) To assess the levels of knowledge and awareness of HIV/AIDS among secondary school students in Eldoret West District.
2) Investigate the students' attitudes to HIV/AIDS and PLWAs.
3) Establish HIV/AIDS prevention methods through practice and behavior.
4) Identify existing cultural practices and misconceptions about HIV/AIDS.
5) Give recommendations on how well HIV/AIDS information can be communicated affectively

Research Questions

1) What do students know about HIV/AIDs infection and transmission rates.
2) What is the attitude of students towards HIV/AIDs and PLWAs
3) How do students prevent themselves from acquiring HIV/AIDS
4) What are the existing cultural practices and misconceptions that enhance the spread of HIV/AIDS
5) How can HIV/AIDS information be affectively communicated to the students.
    "Affective communication is that kind of speaking that touches the feelings and emotions of the listener"

Theoretical Framework

The study is grounded in Harold Lasswells theory of 1948 which has been developed to modern communication theory. This theory is based on mathematical theorems developed by Claude Shannon, an engineer and researcher at Bell Laboratories in 1948. Shannons original theory was later elaborated and given a more popular, non-mathematical formulation by Warren Weaver, a media specialist with the Rockefeller foundation. In effect, Weaver extended Shannons insights about electronic signal transmission and the quantitative measurement of information flows into a broad theoretical model of human communication, which he defined as "all of the ways by which one mind may affect another."

The effectiveness of human communication, Weaver asserted, may be measured by, 'the success with which the meaning conveyed to the receiver leads to the desired conduct on his part.' He thus introduced concepts of human purpose and reaction into what had originally been a set of highly technical equations for analyzing and evaluating transmission of messages. Both mathematical and diagrammatic in character, the Shannon and weaver model measures the efficiency and flexibility of a communication system. It is sometimes referred to as the **S-M-C-R Model**, a mnemonic formula representing the sequence on its main components.

Study Design
The study design was descriptive and cross-sectional and was carried out in the study area between February and March 2010.

Setting
It covered a sample of student population of 405 drawn from 15 out of 45 schools in Eldoret West District. Simple random and probability proportional to size sampling methods were used to sample the schools and the actual participants from each class.
Participants included Students attending secondary schools in the study area in term one 2010.

Study Population
The study was conducted among students attending public secondary schools in Eldoret West District with a population of 3,854 students. The study subjects were drawn from Form One to Form Four students among the sampled schools in the study area.

Those included were:-

a) Students in Form One to Form Four who were present during the study period.

b) All secondary school students in the study area who were willing to join the study by giving informed consent.

Sample size determination

The study covered all secondary schools in Eldoret West District which was curved from the wider Uasin Gishu District, which is situated in the Northern part of Rift Valley Province of Kenya. A sample of 11% of the accessible population was taken. For the questionnaire, this translated into 405 cases of the total 3,854 valid respondents, all students. Eight students were randomly selected from all the schools that took part in the study and took part in Focused Group Discussions (FGDs).

Sampling procedures

This study adopted Mugenda and Mugenda's (1999) multi-stage cluster sampling technique. The schools were first stratified based on Mixed Boarding, Mixed Day, Boy's Boarding, Boy's Day and Girl's Boarding and Day schools. Accordingly, 15 out of 45 schools in the District were sampled. To sample within individual schools, probability proportional to size sampling method was used to allocate sample sizes per class and simple random sampling technique was used in each class to sample the subjects. The student registration numbers were used to obtain a list of computer based random sample. The sample size of 405 students was distributed among these randomly selected schools by using probability proportional to size sampling method. From this calculation, the number assigned for each school was further divided using probability proportional to size sampling technique to fit the distribution of students in these various classes. Eight

6

subjects who participated in FGDs were randomly selected from each school. Two subjects were randomly selected from each form (Forms I-IV) per school. Equal numbers of male and female students were selected from each form in case of mixed schools.

Table 1: Demographics

Variable		Male n (%)	Female n (%)	Total
Gender		207 (51.1)	198 (48.9)	405
School	Urban	135 (33)	130 (32)	265
	Peri-urban	72 (18)	68 (17)	140
Academic form	Form 1	60 (14.8)	61 (15)	121
	Form 2	56 (14)	54 (13)	110
	Form 3	54 (13)	62 (15)	116
	Form 4	37(9)	21 (5)	58
Age group	Less than 14 years	1 (0.25)	0 (0)	1
	14years	8(2)	31(8)	39
	15 years	35 (9)	34 (8)	69
	Above 15 years	162 (40.0)	134 (33.0)	296
Religion	Catholics	50 (12.7)	71 (18)	121
	Protestants	126 (32)	137(34.8)	263
	Muslim	9 (2.2)	12 (3.0)	21

Data collection procedure

Data was collected from the sampled schools between February and March 2010 using self-administered semi-structured, pre-tested questionnaires and FGDs testing on knowledge on a number of variables by the study subjects.

Completed questionnaires were placed in a box next to the exit points for collection by the researcher. The qualitative data was collected from the FGD, with the total number of participants being 8, through use of a structured FGD guide. The FGD was conducted by two trained research assistants: a facilitator and a note taker, and lasted 90 minutes. The session was tape recorded.

Data Analysis

Data from this study was analyzed using SPSS version 15.

Knowledge and awareness on HIV and AIDS/STI

Responses to knowledge questions were classified as correct or incorrect. Then total scores converted to percentages. A score of $\geq$ 70% was considered as very good knowledge, 30-69% was considered as good knowledge and <30% was considered as fair knowledge.

Statistical treatment of data

Descriptive and inferential statistics were used to analyze the collected information. The descriptive statistics used in the data analysis were frequencies, percentages, means, and standard deviation whereas the inferential statistics was the Pearson Product Moment correlation. The percentage means and standard deviation were used for the arrangement of items and answered research questions one, three and four. Pearson Product Moment correlation coefficient was used to determine the relationship between independent (knowledge, attitude, behavioral practices and cultural practices) and dependent variable (HIV/AIDS) and enabled the researcher to respond to research question two.

The collected data by use of the questionnaire was analyzed using the Statistical Package for Social Sciences (SPSS) with the assistance of a statistician. The results obtained were presented in form of tables and charts.

8

The data was transformed through use of cluster weighting technique. The various responses per category were grouped based on their conventional and logical acceptability and suitability. Proportions were compared using the chi square test and statistical significance reported when p-values of less than 0.05 were observed.

Qualitative Data

The tape was transcribed through use of verbatim transcription technique. The transcribed notes and the hand written notes were analyzed qualitatively and were used to dispute or confirm the findings of the quantitative data

Table 2: Distribution of respondents by their sources of information on HIV and AIDS.

Source of information	Frequency	Percentage
School	226	56.0
Church	08	2.0
Radio	28	6.9
Clinic/Hospital/Doctor	47	11.4
Newspaper/Magazine	16	4.0
Public/Posters/Handouts/Brochures	13	3.2
Friends and School Mates	22	5.4
Television	23	5.7
Family members	22	5.4
Total	**405**	**100**

The school was the highest source of information on HIV/AIDs information, followed by the Clinic/Hospital/Doctor then through the radio.

On bivariate analysis it was observed that the source of information was determined by knowledge ($X^2 = 37.488$; df = 24; p = 0.039), risk factors ($X^2 = 49.992$; df = 32; p = 0.022) and type of school ($\mathbf{X^2} = 47.775$; df = 24; p = 0.003).

Discussion

General knowledge and awareness on HIV and AIDS/STI

Accurate knowledge regarding possible routes of transmission is not only critical for decreasing infection rate, it is also important to dispel persistent myths and partial knowledge that can further perpetuate the risk of HIV infection. Lack of knowledge and misconception about HIV and AIDS are key factors in the lack of prevention efforts. Although knowledge alone does not change behaviour, and there is no significant relationship between sexual knowledge and safe sex, it has been shown that knowledge of the facts of HIV transmission plays a role in increasing the likelihood of safe sex through perception of individual risk that mediate action based on knowledge. Three hundred and ninety nine (99%) of the participants were aware about HIV and AIDS. A previous study conducted in western Kenya, Wools et al (1998), reported 96 % awareness, which was much lower. This difference could probably be due to the effects HIV and AIDS awareness campaigns. Awareness on HIV and AIDS among respondents was strongly influenced by their school (X^2 = 47.775; p = 0.003), with respondents in urban schools exhibiting higher awareness levels. This study found that about 245 (60%) of the respondents knew someone who was living with HIV and AIDS. A study in Mozambique showed that (35.7%) of the respondents knew someone with AIDS, whereas in Tanzania, Maswanya et al., (1999) reported (58%) encounter. The Mozambican study also showed that the respondents had multiple sex partners due to lack of encounter with HIV and AIDS patients. Accordingly, it is surmised that lack of encounter with an HIV and AIDS patient may culminate in increased irresponsible sexual behaviour. Consequently, it is inferred that the misconceptions about AIDS may be due to the low level of exposure to people living with HIV and AIDS. This study showed that based on qualitative data, almost all of the groups did not have a clear cut differentiation of HIV and AIDS only one male participant aged fifteen said that AIDS was caused after having the virus weaken the body cells.

11

Approximately 118 (29.2%) of the respondents reported to have had an STI. This was much higher than findings in Mozambique by Ndola *et al* (2006) which showed that only about (18%) of the respondents, had suffered from STIs. These findings were corroborated by FGD results in which participants said that it was a youthful behaviour to engage in sexual acts. However, just about 129(32%) of the study respondents had been tested for HIV. This was far much below expectation, given the high levels of knowledge and awareness on HIV and AIDS. At the same time, majority 364(89.8%) of the respondents reported that HIV patients remained healthy and could transmit the virus. This was much lower than findings by Alene *et al.* (2004) in a study conducted in Ethiopia but higher than findings by Maswanya *et al.* (1999) in Tanzania. About 75(18.5%) of the respondents reported that HIV could be transmitted through a vector. Studies in Kenya by Toroitich-Ruto (2002) have also reported incrimination of vectors in transmission of HIV.

Respondents displayed a wide range of awareness and knowledge on STI, HIV and AIDS. However, the respondents equally often mixed correct information with misconception. This was common in FGDs where some participants reported kissing, mosquito bites and sorcery as possible sources of HIV infection to man. Although they reported knowing that a healthy looking person could be infected with HIV and STIs, some of the participants still said they would rely on outward appearance as a means of identifying those infected with HIV and AIDS. These findings are health threatening as studies in Zambia have shown that respondents who support this view are likely to have a poor risk perception and be more prone to acts of sexual irresponsibility (PSI,2003).

12

Some of the respondents believed that the youth were at a greater risk of infection because of their high levels of sexual activity. However a majority of them thought it was the adults who were at risk because they had been sexually active longer and had more sexual partners. Only a few respondents noted that any one who was sexually active was at risk of HIV infection. Whereas 275 (68%) of the respondents agreed that having safe sex with more than one partner increases ones chances of getting HIV/STI, findings from Tanzania by Maswanya *et al.* Showed that (87.7%) of the respondents felt the same way.

There were no formal HIV and AIDS prevention programmes in any of the sampled schools at the time of this study. The information and awareness messages had been reportedly obtained mainly from the parents, relatives, friends, mass media and other government approved sources. Depending on their level of knowledge and sophistication, family and/or friends may be a source of useful information or may also act as a source of myths, prejudices and misinformation for the youth. Therefore it seemed that the difference between HIV knowledge of the youth in school and all other groups was not related to any particular HIV and AIDS awareness programme. Studies have shown that informing high risk groups of HIV and AIDS requires special informal interventions; so generally, the public awareness programme cannot improve their knowledge significantly. Such HIV and AIDS campaigns have to be realistic, sub-culturally relevant and target specific.

Results

About (99%) indicated that they had heard about AIDS compared to only 4 (1%) who had not. Knowledge had no statistically significant relationship with risk of HIV and AIDS. About 53.3% of the respondents reported to have had sex with males being more likely to have an early sexual debut. Sexual activity was higher among peri-urban respondents (37%) who also had more than 3 sexual partners. About 71.4% of the respondents were willing to change their behaviour to avoid contracting HIV. On bivariate analysis, exposure to risk factors was dependent on gender ($p < 0.05$), perceived risk and condom used were related ($p < 0.05$).

Conclusion

This study concluded that despite their high knowledge and awareness on HIV and AIDS, not all students who were exposed to risk perceived themselves to be at risk. The main preventive method of contracting HIV/AIDS was through condom use, cultural practices like wife inheritance and traditional circumcision increased the risk of infection and that affective communication was not used in schools to reduce HIV/AIDS infection and affection.

Recommendations

The study recommended that though creating more awareness on HIV/AIDs was still necessary to diffuse some misconceptions, more effort was needed to address behavior change among the adolescents especially through affective communication. This can be done through inviting specialized groups to speak to adolescents in schools.

REFERENCES

NASCOP/MoH. *Sentinel Surveillance of HIV and STDs in Kenya.* Nairobi: NASCOP; 2005.

Kamaara, E. K. *"Gender* Relations and Sexual Activity among the Youth and the Role of the church in Kenya"
Doctoral thesis, Eldoret: Moi University, 2003.

Berer M, and Ray S. *Women and HIV/AIDS: An international resource book. information, action and resources on women and HIV/AIDS, reproductive health and sexual relationships.* London (UK): Harper and Collins Publishers, 1993.

NASCOP, *AIDS in Kenya 7th Ed.* Nairobi: NASCOP, 2005.

CBS/MoH/ORC, *Kenya Demographic and Health Survey 2003.* Calverton, Maryland: CBS, MoH and ORC Macro. 2004.

Kermyt GA, and Beutel AM, "HIV/AIDS prevention knowledge among youth in Cape

Town, South Africa." *Journal of Social Sciences* 2007; 3 (3): 143-151.

Fisher A.A, Laing J.E, Stoeckel J E and Townsend J W. *Handbook for family planning operations research designs and sampling 2nd Edition.* New York: Population Council,1998.

Mugenda O, and Mugenda A. *Sample Size Determination; Research methods, Quantitative and Qualitative approaches*, Nairobi: ACTS press; 1999.

Iliyasu Z, Abubakar I.S, Kabir M, and Aliyu MH. "Knowledge of HIV/AIDS and Attitude towards Voluntary Counseling and Testing among Adults in Nigeria." *Journal of the National Medical Association* 2006; 98 (12):24-56.

Babakian T, Freier MC, Hopkins, GL, Diclemente, R, McBride D, Riggs, M. "An Assessment of HIV/AIDS risk in Higher Education Students in Yerevan, Armenia." *AIDS and Behaviour 2004*; 8 (1): 47-61.

Macintyre K, Rutenberg N, Brown B, and Karim A. Understanding Perceptions of HIV risk among Adolescents
in KwaZulu-Natal. AIDS and Behaviour 2004; 8 (3): 237-250.

Wools K.K, Menya D, Muli F, Heilman D, and Jones R. "Perception of Risk, Sexual Behaviour and STD/HIV prevalence in Western Kenya." *East African Medical Journal* 1998; 75 (12):679-691.

Maswanya E, Moji K, Horiguchi I, Nagata K, Aoyagi K, and Takemoto T. "Knowledge, Risk perception of AIDS and reported Sexual Behaviour among Secondary Schools and colleges in Tanzania." *Health Education research* 1999; 14 (2): 185-196.

Ndola P, Leo M, Mazive, E, Vahidnia F, and Strehr M. "Relationship between HIV risk Perception and Condom use: Evidence from a population based survey in Mozambique." *International Family Planning Perspectives.* 2006; 32(4): 192-200.

Alene G. D, Wheeler J. G. and Grosskurth H. "Adolescent Reproductive Health and Awareness of HIV among Rural High School Students, North Western, Ethiopia." *AIDS CARE* 2004; 16 (1): 57-68.

Toroitich-Ruto C. "The effects of HIV/AIDS on Sexual Behaviour of Young People in Kenya. Nairobi. *Family Health International,* 2002; 12(5):34-65.

Population Services International. "Misconceptions, Folk Beliefs, Denial Hinder Risk

Perception among Young Zambian Men. *Research Brief.* 2003.3 (2): 45-67

Pattullo A, "Survey of Knowledge, Behaviour and Attitudes Relating to HIV infection and AIDS among Kenya Secondary School Students." *Family Health International* 1997;4(3): 23-57.

UNAIDS. "AIDS Epidemic Update." Geneva. 2006.

Coates T.J, Reducing High-Risk HIV Behaviours: An Overview of Effective

Approaches. NIH Consensus Development Conference. 1997.

Wrong, L., Chin, C., Low, W., & Jaafar, N. (2009). HIV/AIDS – Related Knowledge Among Malaysian Young Adults: Findings From a Nationwide Survey. *The Medscape Journal of Medicine. : Journal of the International AIDS Society.* Malaysia. Medscape. Retrieved November 17, 2009, from http://www.medscape.com/viewarticle/573213.

Sabastian F Achan 1, Patricia Akweongo 1, Cornelius Debpuur 1 and John Cleland (2009).Coping Strategies of Young Mothers at Risk of HIV/AIDS in the Kassena-Nankana District of Northern Ghana. *African Journal of Reproductive Health Vol 13 No 1* March 2009. http://www.bioline.org.br/pdf?rh09007.

Sarkar N. N (2008). Barriers to condom use. *The European Journal of Contraception & Reproductive Health Care, Volume 13, Issue 2 2008 , pages 114 – 122.* Retrieved on May 23, 2010, from http://www.informaworld.com/smpp/content~content=a791845207&db=all.

Seroney, G. C. (2009). "Knowledge, Attitudes and Practices of Trained Traditional Birth Attendants on HIV AIDS Transmission and Prevention in Kosirai Division, Kenya." A Masters of Nursing Thesis submitted to the Department of Nursing of the School of Health Sciences of the University of Eastern Africa, Baraton.

Tehrani, F.R., and Afzali H. M. (2008) Knowledge, Attitudes and Practices Concerning HIV/AIDS among Iranian at-risk sub-population. *Health Journal, Volume 14, No. 1, January – February, 2008. Pages 1-5.* Retrieved Novemer 19, 2009, from http://www.emro.who.int/Publications/emhj/1401/article16.htm.

TVT (2005) Shame and Secrecy: Genital Mutilation in the US . TVB Daily, Sat Oct 15, 2005 at 12:58:24. Retrieved June 3, 2010, from http://tlctugger.com/Archives/KOS-GenitalIntegrity.htm

UNAIDS (2010). The basic facts about HIV/AIDS SHIV AIDS fact. *UNAIDS.* Retrieved June 3, 2010, from http://www.emro.who.int/sudan/Media/PDF/HIV%20Aids%20Basic%20facts %20Fact%20Sheet%20A%20- %20Sudan%20adapted%205%20Mar%20EDT.pdf

UNESCO (2002). A cultural approach to HIV/AIDS prevention and care: UNESCO/USAID research project. *UNESCO Studies and Reports, Special Series, Issue N°10.* Retrieved May 23, 2010, from http://unesdoc.unesco.org/images/0012/001262/126289e.pdf

UNFPA (2009) Preventing HIV/AIDS among adolescents through integrated communication program. *HIV/AIDS Prevention Among Adolescents: A Global Issue.* UNFPA 220 East 42nd Street New York, NY 10017 USA ISBN #: 0-89714-688-3. Retrieved November, 19 2009, from http://www.unfpa.org/upload/lib_pub_file/224_filename_hiv_adolescents02.p df